Ilia Grohotov
Oleg Oreshaka

Ozone therapy in dentistry

Ilia Grohotov
Oleg Oreshaka

Ozone therapy in dentistry

LAP LAMBERT Academic Publishing

Impressum / Imprint

Bibliografische Information der Deutschen Nationalbibliothek: Die Deutsche Nationalbibliothek verzeichnet diese Publikation in der Deutschen Nationalbibliografie; detaillierte bibliografische Daten sind im Internet über http://dnb.d-nb.de abrufbar.

Alle in diesem Buch genannten Marken und Produktnamen unterliegen warenzeichen-, marken- oder patentrechtlichem Schutz bzw. sind Warenzeichen oder eingetragene Warenzeichen der jeweiligen Inhaber. Die Wiedergabe von Marken, Produktnamen, Gebrauchsnamen, Handelsnamen, Warenbezeichnungen u.s.w. in diesem Werk berechtigt auch ohne besondere Kennzeichnung nicht zu der Annahme, dass solche Namen im Sinne der Warenzeichen- und Markenschutzgesetzgebung als frei zu betrachten wären und daher von jedermann benutzt werden dürften.

Bibliographic information published by the Deutsche Nationalbibliothek: The Deutsche Nationalbibliothek lists this publication in the Deutsche Nationalbibliografie; detailed bibliographic data are available in the Internet at http://dnb.d-nb.de.

Any brand names and product names mentioned in this book are subject to trademark, brand or patent protection and are trademarks or registered trademarks of their respective holders. The use of brand names, product names, common names, trade names, product descriptions etc. even without a particular marking in this works is in no way to be construed to mean that such names may be regarded as unrestricted in respect of trademark and brand protection legislation and could thus be used by anyone.

Coverbild / Cover image: www.ingimage.com

Verlag / Publisher:
LAP LAMBERT Academic Publishing
ist ein Imprint der / is a trademark of
OmniScriptum GmbH & Co. KG
Heinrich-Böcking-Str. 6-8, 66121 Saarbrücken, Deutschland / Germany
Email: info@lap-publishing.com

Herstellung: siehe letzte Seite /
Printed at: see last page
ISBN: 978-3-659-46196-5

Copyright © 2013 OmniScriptum GmbH & Co. KG
Alle Rechte vorbehalten. / All rights reserved. Saarbrücken 2013

Ozone therapy in dentistry

Performed by: Grohotov I. O.

The supervisor: MD, prof. Oreshaka O. V.

Table of contents

1. Introduction..3
2. History of ozone therapy..6
3. Biological and clinical effects of ozone.........................9
4. General contraindications..15
5. Ozone in dentistry..17
6. Conclusion..49
7. References..50

Introduction.

At present, more and more persistently shown interest in drug-free treatment that can replace or significantly limit the need for drugs and thus affect various aspects of the pathological process, contribute to the regulation of disturbed homeostasis, improve the functional status of the various organs and systems that enhance the body's defenses. One of these methods is the therapeutic use of ozone for receiving considerable spread in our country and abroad. In recent years, due to a number of international congresses and conferences it is possible to generalize the accumulated considerable experimental and clinical data concerning the use of ozone, the indications and contraindications for the purpose of the ground to determine the methods of use of ozone and clarify the parameters of specific therapeutic techniques.

Wide use of ozone for the treatment and prevention showed its clinical efficacy, good tolerability, the relative cheapness of the method, and therefore significantly cheaper - all contribute to the fact that ozone therapy in isolation or combined with other medical factors should be widely used in clinics and hospitals.

It is distressing to note that often ozone therapists are more interested in simply knowing the ozone dosage rather than to understand how ozone acts and why we can avoid toxicity [58]. This behavior reveals a lack of knowledge of the fundamental bases regulating a judicious use of ozone and is the result of a superficial preparation acquired during an occasional ozone therapy's course of a few hours. This is not surprising because during the last three decades, on the basis of Wolff's suggestion, ozone therapy has been used by practitioners in Europe in an empirical fashion. Unfortunately, even today, most ozone therapists have either a misconception or know only a few technical tips for performing ozone therapy. This problem, associated with the difficulties and cost of performing extensive clinical studies, has hindered real progress, and ozone therapy remains a scarcely known and objected complementary practice. Worst of all, in some countries, often without any medical qualification, quacks continue to inject either ozone intravenously, a procedure prohibited since 1984 in Germany because of the risk of pulmonary embolism and death, or ozonated saline containing a certain toxic amount of hypochloric acid. Moreover, a distinguished American chemist has affirmed the dogma that "ozone is toxic any way you deal with it," reinforcing the concept that ozone should never be used in medicine. This situation has generated a sort of crusade against ozone therapy in spite of the fact that ozone is considered one of the best disinfectants capable of preventing infection outbreaks. This is becoming a crucial advantage because critically ill patients acquire infections while in hospitals and a number of them die every year as a result.

During the last 14 years, we have made a great effort to examine ozone therapy in a scientific fashion both at a basic and clinical level, and we now have some ideas how ozone acts, how and why its toxicity can be controlled and how therapeutic effects can be exerted. There is no need to invoke philosophical speculations because the mechanisms of action are in the realm of classical biochemistry, physiology and pharmacology. This review aims to give the reader the essential information about using ozone in general medicine and dentistry.

History of ozone therapy.

The German chemist Christian Friedrich Schönbein (1840), of the University of Basel in Switzerland is regarded as the Father of ozone therapy. When he passed an electrical discharge through water, a gas strange smell was produced, which he called Ozone, derived from the Greek word ozein which means odor. In 1857 Joachim Hänsler, a German physicist and physician, along with German physician, Hans Wolff, developed the first ozone generator for medical use. Dr. C. Lender in 1870, for the first time applied O3 into medical field. He purified blood in test tubes by using O3. Later, O3 application gained as a popularity as a therapeutic procedure throughout Europe and America. In 1881, it was used as a disinfectant in the treatment of diphtheria. Dr. Charles Kenworthy, a Florida physician, in 1885, published his experiences with ozone in the Florida Medical Association Journal. In October 1893, Ousbaden, Holland became the first city to utilize a water treatment plant using ozone. In World War I and II it was used to treat wounded soldiers in the trenches. In early 20th century Food and Drug Act, revised its use and effect in the field of medicine. They considered it as perfectly legal to use in US. Since then, it was used in the treatment of then deadly diseases such as tuberculosis, pneumonia, diabetes etc. It was also used to cure wounds, gangrene and the effects of poisonous gas. As of 1929, more than 114 diseases were listed for treatment with oxygen/ozone therapy. A German dentist, Dr. E.A. Fisch, in 1950 was the first dentist to use ozone on regular basis in his dental practice in Zurich, Switzerland and published numerous papers on its application. He used ozone to treat Ernst Payr, a renowned Austrian surgeon, who then became an ozone enthusiast and began a line of research dedicated to its use in healthcare. At that time, ozone therapy was difficult and limited due to the lack of ozone-resistant materials, such as Nylon, Dacron and Teflon, until when ozone-resistant materials were manufactured. Beginning of dental-application research with the approval of an Institutional Review Board for Human Research from Capital University of Integrative Medicine in Washington, D.C., started in 2001. The first formal lecture on oxygen/ozone therapy was given in 2001 at Capital University. Later on, extensive research continued with the publication of Dr. Siegfried Rilling's and Dr. Renate Viebahn's text, "The Use of Ozone in Medicine." This text was a standard until 2002, when Dr. Velio Bocci published "Oxygen/Ozone Therapy – A Critical Review." This was followed by first dental-applications clinical seminar in Louisville, Ky., in 2003. In 2004, Professor Edward Lynch of Belfast, United Kingdom, contributed to and edited the book "Ozone: The Revolution in Dentistry." Numerous researchers since that time have worked to elucidate the nature and actions of ozone.

In Russia the main development center of ozone therapy is located in Nizhny Novgorod, where the most famous russian scientists of this field of knowledge worked. In 1977 such knew method as intravenous injection of ozonated solutions was developed. In 1986 first carried ozonized cardiopulmonary bypass in cardiac surgery was used. In 1992 the russian association of ozone therapists was created and since that knew technologies and equipment has been discovered. Thanks to the emergence of a new generation of medical ozone generators in medicine we have an ability to use strictly controlled ozone concentrations in practically all fields of medicine, including dentistry [1,55].

Biological and clinical effects of ozone.

The ozonation process is therefore characterized by the formation of ROS and LOPs acting in two phases. This process happens either ex vivo (as a typical example in the blood collected in a glass bottle) or in vivo (after an intramuscular injection of ozone) but, while ROS are acting immediately and disappear (early and short-acting messengers), LOPs, via the circulation, distribute throughout the tissues and eventually only a few molecules bind to cell receptors.

Their pharmacodynamics allows minimizing their potential toxicity and allows them to become late and long-lasting messengers. Formation of ROS in the plasma is extremely rapid and is accompanied by a transitory and small ozone dose dependent decrease (ranging from 5 to 25%) of the antioxidant capacity. Importantly, this return to normal within 15–20 min owes to the efficient recycling of oxidized compounds such as dehydroascorbate to ascorbic acid. H_2O_2 diffuses easily from the plasma into the cells and its sudden appearance in the cytoplasm represents the triggering stimulus: depending upon the cell type, different biochemical pathways can be concurrently activated in erythrocytes, leukocytes and platelets resulting in numerous biological effects. The rapid reduction to water is operated by the high concentration of GSH, CAT and GSH-Px; nonetheless, H_2O_2 must be above the threshold concentration for activating several biochemical pathways. LOPs act as repeated stressors on the bone marrow and these frequent stimuli cause the adaptation to the ozone stress during erythrogenesis with upregulation of antioxidant enzymes. Once again, the crucial messenger is hydrogen peroxide, which after entering into the cytoplasm of blood mononuclear cells (BMC) by oxidizing selected cysteines, activates a tyrosine kinase, which then phosphorylates the transcription factor nuclear factor kB, allowing the release of a heterodimer (p50lp65). This complex moves on to the nucleus and switches on some hundred genes eventually responsible for causing the synthesis of several proteins, among which are the acute-phase reactants and numerous interleukins.

Clinical effects of ozone therapy

Depending on the concentration and means of administration of ozone distinguish the following effects provided by ozone on the body:

1. *Antibacterial, antifungal and antiviral*

When applied topically in the form of a gas mixture or ozonated solutions possible to use high concentrations of ozone, which have direct effects on oxidative membrane of microorganisms. Ozone kills virtually all species of bacteria, fungi, viruses and protozoa. This gram positive bacteria and viruses capsular having lipid bilayer, are particularly susceptible to oxidation. Introduction therapeutic concentrations of ozone in the body causes bactericidal an effect that is mediated by the activation of non-specific defense system (activation of phagocytosis, increased synthesis of cytokines - interferon, tumor -necrotizing factor, interleukins), and cellular components and humoral immunity, known data on the partial oxidation of receptors for viruses, which makes them incapable of binding to viruses. Also revealed inhibition of the enzyme reverse transcriptase.

2. The anti-inflammatory effect.

Ozone is the ability oxidizing the compound containing double bonds, in particular arachidonic acid (20, 4) and prostaglandins are formed from it – biologically active substances involved in the development and maintenance of inflammatory process. Furthermore, ozone recovers metabolic reactions in tissues the site of inflammation and corrects the pH of the oxidation of the double bonds in other (purely pathological) compounds formed from arachidonic acid- Leukotrienes - partly due to the effectiveness of ozone therapy in bronchial asthma.

3. Analgesic effect

Due to ozone on the one hand oxidation degradation products of protein molecules, so-called algopeptidov affecting the nerve endings in the damaged tissue and determining the intensity of pain response, on the other hand, normalization of the antioxidant system and accordingly decrease the amount of toxic molecular peroxidation products lipids in cell membranes that alter function membranovstroennyh enzymes involved in the synthesis of ATP and maintaining life of tissues and organs [56].

4. Detoxification effect of ozone appears to be corrected and metabolic activation in the liver and kidneys, which provides the performance of a core function - neutralization and excretion of toxic compounds.

5. Activation of oxygen-dependent processes.

The introduction of even very low doses of ozone accompanied by an increase in blood free and dissolved oxygen. Observed rapid intensification of enzymes catalyze the aerobic oxidation of carbohydrates, lipids and proteins formation energy substrate ATP. Very important is the activation of the enzyme mitochondrial H-ATPase determining conjugation processes of respiration and oxidative phosphorylation, which is a result of the synthesis of ATP.

6. Optimization of pro-and antioxidant systems of the body.

It is one of the main biological effects of systemic exposure to ozone therapy, implemented through the influence on the cell membrane and is to normalize the balance of the levels of peroxide lipid and antioxidant protection. In response to the introduction ozone in the tissues and organs compensatory increase occurs primarily the activity of antioxidant enzymes superoxide dismutase (SOD), catalase and glutathione peroxidase. Due to the recovery of aerobic metabolic reactions and accumulate NADN2 NADFN2 that are proton donors to restore oxidized components non-enzymatic antioxidant system (glutathione, vitamin E, ascorbic acid, etc.). The use of exogenous antioxidants to preliminary calculations appointed dose is required when used high concentrations of ozone.

7. The haemostatic effect of ozone is dose dependent. High concentrations assigned when applied externally to cause pronounced hypercoagulable effect. Parenteral administration of low ozone concentrations, in contrast, is characterized by a decrease in platelet and coagulation components of hemostasis and increased fibrinolytic activity.

8. Immunomodulatory properties of ozone are based on its interaction with lipid membranes of cell structures and the conditions. Low concentrations of ozone contribute accumulation on the membrane of phagocytic cells, monocytes and macrophages hydrophilic compounds - ozonides that stimulate the synthesis of these cells of various classes of cytokines. Cytokines, being biologically activity of the peptide contributes to further activation of nonspecific protection system (increased body temperature, the development of liver proteins acute phase) and, in addition, activated cellular and humoral immunity. All together contributes to the treatment of secondary immunodeficiencies.

Before starting to describe the use of ozone in dentistry it will be useful to say a few words about the application of ozone in medicine generally.

Topical Ozone Applications in general medicine

In the local application of an O3/O2 gas mixture externally to the skin or to wounds, already practiced during the First World War, it was the disinfectant and deodorizing effect of ozone that stood in the foreground. It is now known that, with the topical application of O3/O2 gas mixtures, from ozonized water or ozone cream (ozonides) and beyond, a wound healing effect is produced which is being made use of to an increasingly successful extent.

Indications

§ External ulcers (ulcus cruris, decubitus ulcers)
§ Burns, superinfected
§ Skin lesions (wounds)
§ Local infections (smear infections, herpes simplex, herpes zoster, mycosis)
§ Eye injuries and infections.

Application forms

§ Ozonized water (acute treatment: e.g. injuries, burns, ulcers, as intraoperative
rinsing)
§ Pressure-free application in ozone-resistant plastic bags, in the form of transcutaneous O3 rinsing (e.g. ulcus cruris, immune vasculitis)
§ Subatmospheric ozone gas application under an ozone-resistant suction cup (e.g. decubitus)
§ O3 gas application in the low-pressure plastic boot ("Rokitansky boot") (e.g. diabetic gangrene)
§ Ozone cream (ozonides) for long-term treatment: e.g. lesions, burns [12].

General contraindications.

Ozone therapy is a well established alternative and complementary therapy in most mainland European countries where health authorities have tolerated such practice. The European Cooperation of Medical Ozone Societies, founded in 1972, publishes guidelines on medical indications and contraindications of ozone and hosts training seminars. Physicians can legally use ozone treatments in their practice without fear of prosecution.

Technology of ozone therapy are also used in medicine such as oncology section. Found that low concentrations of ozone in cancer patients have immunomodulatory effect, which increases the effectiveness of anti-tumor activity of cytotoxic drugs [6].

Conserning about ozone toxicity we can present the results of well-known study of german scientists, were Jacobs analyzed side effects occurring in over 5 million ozone therapy sessions in 384775 patients. Technical errors accounted for minor problems in a minute percentage (0,00007%) of patients – one of the lowest in medicine [17].

Nevertheless, the following are contraindications for use of ozone therapy:

- Pregnancy
- Glucose-6-phosphate-dehydrogenase deficiency (favism)
- Hyperthyroidism
- Severe anemia
- Severe myasthenia

- Active hemorrhage
- Acute alcohol intoxication
- Recent Myocardial infarction

Ozone therapy in dentistry.

Ozone, an allotropic form of oxygen, is successfully used in the treatment of different diseases for more than a hundred years. It is highly valued for various effects, such as antimicrobial, antihypoxic, analgesic, immunostimulating etc. on biological systems. These mechanisms of action supported with a lot of case reports and scientific studies allow using it in different fields of medicine. This review of literature is another attempt to summarize different modalities of ozone application in dentistry. Further studies are necessary to standardize indications and treatment protocols of this promising medical agent.

The main use of ozone in dentistry is relays on its antimicrobial properties. It is proved to be effective against both Gram positive and Gram negative bacteria, viruses and fungi [10].

According to German dentist Fritz Kramer, ozone, such as in the form of ozonated water, can be used in the following ways.

1. as a powerful disinfectant

2. in its ability to control bleeding

3. in its ability to cleanse wounds in bones and soft tissues.

4. by increasing the local supply of oxygen to the wound area, ozone can improve healing.

5. ozonated water can increase temperature in the area of the wound, and this increase the metabolic processes related to wound healing.

Dr. Kramer points out that ozonated water can be used in a number of different ways:

1. as a mouth rinse (especially in cases of gingivitis, periodontitis, or stomatitis);

2. as a spray to cleanse the affected area, and to disinfect oral mucosa, cavities and in general dental surgery;

3. as an ozone/water jet to clean cavities of teeth being capped, receiving root canal therapy, and in treating painful gingivitis and stomatitis.

Appliances producing ozone for dental use

1. HealOzone by KaVo is air-based and the application of the gas takes place in a closed circuit. Its surplus is sucked out and neutralized by manganese ions. The concentration of ozone in the cap adjacent to the tissue amounts to 2100 ppm. Perfect air tightness of the cap is necessary for the application of ozone. Therefore, the application is only possible on the surfaces where such air tightness can be provided.

2. OzonyTron by MYMED Gmb H. - Oxygen activation generator (OzonytronX—Biozonix, München, Germany) uses the power of high frequency and voltage. Activated oxygen (ozone) concentration can be adjusted in 5 levels via current strength. Inside the glass probe, which is formed by a double glass camera, is a noble gasses mixture that is conducting and emitting electromagnetic energy. When the tip of the probe gets in contact with the body it emits energy around the treated area and splits environmental diatomic oxygen in singular atomic oxygen and ozone. The concentration of ozone in the operation field is 10 to 100 µg/ml (becomes a fungi-, viru-, and bactericide at the intensity of 1–5 µg/ml). There is no closed circuit here, therefore, ozone can be applied to the places that are difficult to reach, e.g. gingival pockets or root canals.

3. Product photo (Prozone) by W&H - It is characterized by its ease of use and safety of application (preset tissue-compatible dosages in the indication areas of periodontitis and endodontitis). Prozone ensures a hygienic procedure during the gassing of the pockets due to its exchangeable plastic attachments (Perio tips or Endo tips).

A few words should be said about the use of ozone to sterilize dental equipment. Ozone tool penetrates not only kill viruses, fungi and bacteria, but without damaging the material. Therefore, there is no need to use chemicals, steam or heat. Also, lower concentrations of ozone can be used for processing work surfaces in dental offices [29].

Now we'll try to describe the main ways of use of ozone in clinical dentistry based on scientific data and our clinical experience.

Muller et al. compared the influence of ozone gas with photodynamic therapy (PDT) and known antiseptic agents (2% Chlorhexidine, 0,5 and 5% hypochlorite solutions) on a multispecies oral biofilm in vitro. The following bacteria were studied – Actinomyces naeslundii, Veillonella dispar, Fusobacterium nucleatum, Streptococcus sobrinus, Streptococcus oralis and Candida albicans. Gasiform ozone was produced by vacuum ozone delivery system Kavo Healozone.
They concluded that the matrix-embedded microbial populations in biofilm are well protected towards antimicrobial agents. Only 5 %

Hypochlorite solution was able to eliminate all bacteria effectively. Usage of gasiform ozone or PDT was not able to reduce significantly or completely eliminate bacteria in the biofilm.

Interest to practical endodontists, in our opinion, may preconstitute a new unit of the company Apoza "OzoneDTA". Proposed for this purpose apparatus "OzoneDTA" is not only the ozone generator. Application of this apparatus is based on a combination of ozone action and contact darsonvalizatsii. thanks darsonvalizatsii is arterial vasodilation and venous level, accelerating etsya microcirculation, increased delivery of nutrients, as well as activation of metabolic processes in the tissues. The main properties of ozone, which formed in the machine and fed via conical tip, it is necessary to carry the following: bactericidal and antiviral (due to high oxidative the ability of ozone destroys skin microbial cells, acting DNA and RNA viruses and bacteria). thanks to a combination of actions and darsonvalizatsii ozone "OzoneDTA" achieved a number of presents: a high disinfectant effect, accelerating tissue regeneration, that avoids the use of antibiotics in the treatment, acting only on the area of interventions [33].

The research results also show the high efficiency of ozone in the treatment of dental caries. In the case of shallow cavities of ozone used for the treatment of tooth surfaces with reuse remineralizing solution. In case of deep cavities damaged dentine after treatment applied composite filling materials. It is important to note, that ozone did not significantly affect the dentin bond strength of a silorane-based resin composites [4,20,35].

In preventive dentistry ozone treatment either alone or combined with a re-mineralizing solution was found to be effective for remineralization of initial fissure caries lesions [5]. Also it can be effectively combined with the fissure sealants in pediatric dentistry. The treatment of the enamel with KaVo HealOzone after etching does not affect either microleakage or penetration proportion of flowable composite or sealing resin. There is no statistically significant difference in a degree of penetration between different groups of sealing materials. Groups of materials with flowable composite in combination with an adhesive system show a good degree of penetration into the fissure and low microleakage meaning that they can be used as a fissure sealing materials [28]. Ozonated water strongly inhibited the accumulation of experimental dental plaque in vitro. After the dental plaque samples from human subjects were exposed to ozonated water in vitro, almost no viable bacterial cells were detected. These results suggest that ozonated water should be useful in reducing the infections caused by oral microorganisms in dental plaque [60].

There is a well-known effect of an ozone delivery system (HealOzone; KaVo, Biberach, Germany) in reducing dentin hypersensitivity. An 8-week, 3-visit, triple-blinded, randomized controlled clinical trial with 2 HealOzone machines (ozone/air) involving 44 subjects was conducted. The pain in response to tactile stimulus or desiccation was assessed by using a 100-mm visual analogue scale. Also, the global subjects' perception of sensitivity was assessed at each visit by using the visual analogue scale. No subjects reported an increase in pain or any adverse effect. All subjects reported a clinically significant reduction of pain at each follow-up relative to baseline; however, the difference between the study groups was not statistically significant. The effect of treatment of hypersensitive teeth with ozone reduces the pain sensation, but this effect cannot be distinguished from the placebo treatment [8,23,40].

Besrukova and others [16] studied the comparative antimicrobial activity of ozone-oxygen mixture in respect of a mixed culture of the root canal with chronic periodontitis. It is noted that when the ozone concentration of 40 mg / ml is determined by complete inhibition of growth of pathogenic microorganisms.

Holmes J. [44] assessed antimicrobial effect of Kavo Healozone device on primary root caries lesions (PRCL) and evaluated the efficiency of ozone. As a result, ozone exposure to either 10 or 20 s under experimental conditions reduced the total levels of micro-organisms in the PRCLs to < 1% of the control values. So, leathery non cavitated primary root caries can be arrested non-operatively with ozone and remineralizing products. Initial studies have indicated that an application of ozone for a period of either 10 or 20 seconds is capable of clinically reversing leathery root carious lesions. It is suggested that, subject to confirmation from extensive trials, this simple and non-invasive technique may benefit many patients with root caries throughout the world since this approach to treat root caries can easily be employed in primary care clinics and in the domiciliary treatment of home-bound elderly people and immobile patients in hospices and hospitals [9,11].

In endodontic ozone is one of the most effective disinfectants [37]. For example, biofilms of resistant species such as Enterococcus faecalis pose a major challenge in the treatment of root canals with established periapical disease. In the study Case and others examined the effects of gaseous ozone delivered into saline on biofilms of E. faecalis in root canals of extracted teeth with and without the use of passive ultrasonic agitation. Analysis revealed that 1% sodium hypochlorite was the most effective disinfecting agent followed by ozone combined with ultrasonic agitation, ozone alone, and finally ultrasonic alone. Although none of the treatment regimes were able to reliably render canals sterile under the conditions used, ozone gas delivered into irrigating fluids in the root canal may be useful as an adjunct for endodontic disinfection [21].

Sevi and others studied antibacterial effect of Kavo Healozone device on Streptococcus mutans in comparison with the already proven activity of two dentin-bonding systems. Their findings show that an 80 s application of ozone is a very promising therapy for elimination of residual micro-organisms in deep cavities and therefore of potentially increasing the clinical success of restorations. Also ozone treatment prior to bracket bonding does not affect the shear bond strength. The tests also showed no statistically significant difference whether the superficial decayed dentine had been removed before ozone or with chlorhexidine treatment or not. It can be concluded that gaseous ozone or chlorhexidine gel application for 30 s to deep occlusal carious cavities had no significant immediate antimicrobial effects whether the superficial decayed layers dentine were removed or not [42].

Nagayoshi et al. tested the efficacy of ozonated water on survival and permeability of oral micro-organisms and dental plaque. They confirm that ozonated water (0.5–4 mg/l) was highly effective in killing of both gram positive and gram negative micro-organisms.

Furthermore ozonated water had strong bactericidal activity against bacteria in plaque biofilm, which can be proved also by that fact that ozone application was found to remove the toothbrushes bristles microbiota following conventional brushing. Maximum decontamination efficacy of ozone treatment was observed after 30 min while exposure for short time periods seems to be inefficient which probably reflect the low dose of ozone used in this study [13].

In addition, ozonated water inhibited the accumulation of experimental dental plaque in vitro. High-concentrated gaseous and aqueous ozone was dose-, strain- and time-dependently effective against the tested microorganisms in suspension and the biofilm test model [48]. This preliminary study has shown that the infusion of ozone into non-carious dentine prevented biofilm formation in vitro from S. mutans and L. acidophilus over a four-week period. The possibility exists that ozone treatment may alter the surface wettability of dentine through reaction with organic constituents [52].

Ozonized water applied on a daily basis can accelerate the healing rate in oral mucosa. The comparison with wounds without treatment shows that daily treatment with ozonized water accelerates the physiological healing rate.

It remains unclear why ozonized water has this accelerating effect on wound healing. Diverse biological effects have been observed with application of ozone. The microbiological properties should be noted, these being clearly more accentuated in solution than in a dry ozone-air mixture. The wound receives more oxygen when ozonized water is applied. The modification of wound healing under application of oxygen is well known: the shortening of initial wound healing time, the enhancement of phagocytes activity defending cells, the accelerated migration of epithelial cells, the activation of fibroblasts and the importance for collagen synthesis are some important examples. It should be noted that the influence of ozone leads to a higher expression of cytokines that are important for wound healing, especially TGF-β1, an important substance for regulation and coordination in the initial wound healing phase. TGF-β1 has a marked influence on cell proliferation, chemotaxis (monocytes and fibroblasts), angiogenesis, synthesis of extracellular matrix and collagen synthesis. Large studies performed in vitro and in vivo have showed that TGF-β1 leads to a pronounced acceleration of wound healing. One single application leads to clearly visible effects. This application though, must be performed immediately; 24 hours postoperatively the positive effect is completely lost [31].

Huth studied the effect of ozone on non-cavitated fissure carious lesions in permanent molars. After 3 months, explorative data analysis revealed that the ozone-treated lesions showed significantly more caries reversal or reduced caries progression than the untreated control lesions within the group of patients at high current caries risk (Wilcoxon-Test, P= 0.035). There was no statistical significance examining the whole study population. From the data it can be concluded that ozone application significantly improved non-cavitated initial fissure caries in patients at high caries risk over a 3-month period. Also aqueous ozone revealed the highest level of biocompatibility of the tested antiseptics [45,46].

Maybe the most impressive results were gained in periodontology, were ozonetherapy is now widely using. Clinical and laboratory studies of the effectiveness of ozone therapy showed that treatment with ozone-oxygen mixture is a qualitatively new solution for actual problems of the treatment of periodontal disease.

Indications for use of ozone in Periodontology:
-Catarrhal gingivitis
- Necrotizing ulcerative gingivitis
- Chronic periodontitis
- Rapidly forms of periodontitis.
Thus, the following methods of ozone application in cancer patients:
- External exposure (ozone-oxygen mixture ozonized water solutions, ozonized vegetable oils)
- Submucosal injection of ozonated saline.

Ebensberger et al. evaluated the effect of irrigation with ozonated water on the proliferation of cells in the periodontal ligament adhering to the root surfaces of 23 freshly extracted completely erupted third molars. The teeth were randomly treated by intensive irrigation with ozonated water for 2 min or irrigation with a sterile isotonic saline solution, serving as a control group. The periodontal cells of these teeth were studied immunohistochemically to mark proliferating cell nuclear antigen (PCNA). It was observed that the labeling index (the number of positive cells compared to the total number of cells suggesting enhancement of metabolism) was higher among the teeth irrigated with ozone (7.8% vs. 6.6%); however, the difference was not statistically significant ($p = 0.24$). They concluded that the 2 min irrigation of the avulsed teeth with non-isotonic ozonated water might lead not only to a mechanical cleansing, but also decontaminate the root surface, with no negative effect on periodontal cells remaining on the tooth surface.

Nagayoshi et al. tested the efficacy of three different concentrations of ozone water (0.5, 2, and 4 mg/ml in distilled water) on the time-dependent inactivation of cariogenic, periodontopathogenic and endodontopathogenic microbes (Streptococcus, Porphyromonas gingivalis and endodontalis, Actinomyces actinomycetemcomitans, Candida albicans) in culture and in biofilms. They confirm that ozonated water was highly effective in killing of both gram positive and gram negative micro-organisms.

Depending on the dosage, the oral microbes were inactivated after 10 seconds. Gram negative anaerobes, such as Porphyromonas endodontalis and Porphyromonas gingivalis were substantially more sensitive to ozonated water than gram positive oral streptococci and Candida albicans in pure culture. Furthermore ozonated water had strong bactericidal activity against bacteria in plaque biofilm. In addition, ozonated water inhibited the accumulation of experimental dental plaque in vitro.

Ramzy et al. irrigated the periodontal pockets by ozonized water in 22 patients suffering from aggressive periodontitis (age range from 13 to 25 years). Periodontal pockets were irrigated with 150 ml of ozonized water over 5 to 10 minutes once weekly, for a clinical four weeks study, using a blunt tipped sterile plastic syringe. High significant improvement regarding pocket depth, plaque index, gingival index and bacterial count was recorded related to quadrants treated by scaling and root planning together with ozone application. They also reported significant reduction in bacterial count in sites treated with ozonized water.

Huth et al. in their study declared that the aqueous form of ozone, as a potential antiseptic agent, showed less cytotoxicity than gaseous ozone or established antimicrobials (chlorhexidine digluconate-CHX 2%, 0.2%; sodium hypochlorite-NaOCl 5.25%, 2.25%; hydrogen peroxide-H_2O_2 3%) under most conditions. Therefore, aqueous ozone fulfils optimal cell biological characteristics in terms of biocompatibility for oral application.

Kronusová used ozone in following cases: prevention of dental caries in fissures of the first permanent molars in children, application of ozone in prepared cavity, after tooth extraction, in case of postextractional complications, in patients with chronic gingivitis, periodontitis and periodontal abscesses, herpes labialis, purulent periodontitis, dentition difficilis, etc. Almost all patients with gingivitis showed subjective and objective improvement of their status, as well as patients with periodontal abscess, where no exudation was observed. Application of ozone after tooth extraction was found also quite useful – only 10 % of patients suffered from such complication as alveolitis sicca, but even in these cases the clinical course was shorter and more moderate.

Kshitish and Laxman conducted a randomized, double-blind, crossover split-mouth study on 16 patients suffering from generalized chronic periodontitis. The study period of 18 days was divided into two time-intervals, i.e. baseline (0 days) to 7th day, with a washout period of 4 days followed by a second time interval of 7 days.

Subgingival irrigation of each half of the mouth with either ozone or chlorhexidine was done at different time intervals. They observed a higher percentage of reduction in plaque index (12%), gingival index (29%) and bleeding index (26%) using ozone irrigation as compared to chlorhexidine. The percentile reduction of Aa (25%) using ozone was appreciable as compared to no change in Aa occurrence using chlorhexidine. By using O_3 and chlorhexidine, there was no antibacterial effect on *Porphyromonas gingivalis* (Pg) and *Tannerella forsythensis*. The antifungal effect of ozone from baseline (37%) to 7th day (12.5%) was pronounced during the study period, unlike CHX, which did not demonstrate any antifungal effect. No antiviral property of ozone was observed. The antiviral efficacy of chlorhexidine was better than that of ozone. They concluded that despite the substantivity of chlorhexidine, the single irrigation of ozone is quite effective to inactivate microorganisms.

When using ozonated solutions ozone concentration is determined by the choice of the degree of severity of inflammation in periodontal tissues. In a case of active inflammation it is necessary to use ozonated saline solution with a high concentration of ozone in the ozone-air mixture; it is carried out by the following procedure:
- Rinse the mouth with an ozonated solution 2 times a day for 10-14 days
- Irrigation of periodontal pockets from the syringe for 5-10 minutes 8-10 times.
When reducing the activity of the inflammatory process or the chronic course of ozone therapy is used to influence the resistance of the oral cavity and improve the processes of regeneration:
- Rinse mouth ozonated saline for 5 days with a low concentration of ozone in the ozone-air mixture 1500-2000 mg / ml
- Application of ozonized olive oil (the concentration of ozone in the ozone-air mixture 3500-4000 mcg / ml) for 30 minutes two times a day, for 5 days [15].

Also effective is the use of ozone therapy in degenerative pathology of periodontal tissue on a background of severe tissue hypoxia [57]. Forms of use:

- Intravenous infusions of ozonated saline solution
- Rinse mouth ozonized water solutions with ozone concentration 1.5-8 mg / ml
- Application of ozonated oils.

The data obtained by microbiogical investigation, evidence-out that the use of a scattered considered non-drug methods does not achieve the required effect in the treatment of chronic generation a localized periodontitis. This is limited exposure to the applicable therapy for one of the pathogenesis factors- Or a microorganism or a non-specific protection of microorganism. Integrated application of laser radiation and ozone therapy achieves clinical effect on long-term. Thus ozone suppressing anaerobic microorganisms that have an adverse effect in respect SRI normal flora of the oral cavity. A laser beam is an important link in the stimulation of local factors nonspecific protection [32].

Effective is the use of ozone therapy after conducting professional oral hygiene. It is known that the mechanical removal of plaque does not remove parodontopatogenic bacteria. But the use of ozone significantly reduces the concentration of microorganisms and creates favorable conditions for the subsequent healing [25].

A single subgingival irrigation of 0.01 mg l(-1) ozonated water can effectively reduce the gingival inflammation in orthodontic patients, which is also reflected in the reduction of LDH enzyme levels. However, further randomized controlled trials are required to validate the use of ozone irrigation in orthodontic patients for plaque control measures [27].

Interesting are the results of studies on the use of ozone therapy in such a complex disease as glossodiniya. In this case, the authors used the following method: intravenous drip infusions of ozonated saline solution with a concentration of ozone generated by the ozone-oxygen mixture 1200 mcg / mL. The course of treatment was u-8 procedures and by the end of the course most of the patients reported increased efficiency, improve overall health, emotional stability of the state. In general, the inclusion of ozone therapy in a comprehensive treatment plan glossodinii allowed to increase its efficiency by 29% [51].

Despite the advantages that the therapeutic use of ozone offers, reservations remain in terms of its application in the oral and maxillofacial area [78]. In surgical dentistry ozone or its products can be used to influence bone density and the quality of dental implant osseointegration. Therefore, topically applied ozonated oil may influence bone density and the quality of osseointegration around dental implants [30]. Gaseous ozone showed selective efficacy to reduce adherent bacteria on titanium and zirconia without affecting adhesion and proliferation of osteoblastic cells [43].

In extractive surgery ozone is indicated for the prevention of postoperative complications. For instance, it is certain that oral extractive surgery is a remarkable trigger to avascular osteonecrosis of the jaw in patients treated with pyrophosphate analogous. The object of the study of Agrillo and others was to demonstrate how dental extraction becomes possible in a patient with avascular bisphosphonate-related jaw osteonecrosis or in those who simply received pyrophosphate analogous when proper treatment with ozone therapy has been done [2].

Intuitively, ozone therapy is very useful in both acute and chronic bacterial, viral and fungi infections because the generated ROS are the natural and most effective agents to which even antibiotic resistant pathogens do not resist. Moreover, improvement of metabolism and immunological functions contribute to a favorable outcome. Abscesses, anal fissures, fistulae, bed sores, furunculosis, inveterate osteomyelitis, vulvovaginitis, necrotizing fasciitis and torpid ulcers of various origin have been shown to improve rapidly, particularly using the combination of O3-AHT with topical treatment using either direct O_2_ O_3 exposure or the cleansing and stimulating effect of ozonated water and oil. The activity of ozonated solutions in eliminating the infectivity and enhancing healing is almost unbelievable. However, in Western countries accustomed to the use of antibiotic creams (often with corticosteroids) there is no mental attitude to profitably use the inexpensive and most active ozonated oil [18].

The methods of treatment of patients with acute inflammatory processes of the maxillofacial region: it is shown that the positive effects of ozone therapy in the treatment of abscesses and abscesses is to reduce the level of endogenous intoxication, normalization of free radical oxidation, the local resistance of the mouth. The stimulatory effect of ozone is manifested not only in acute inflammatory processes, but also in the low-intensity chronic diseases (osteomyelitis, chronic abscesses) [14]. Turning to the program integrated patients with fractures jaws reduces the concentration of ozone therapy microbes in the oral fluid, which leads to a reduction of inflammatory complications percent more than 2 times [73]. The results suggest that odontoblastic cells exhibit inflammatory responses against LPS and that ozonated water has the ability to improve LPS-induced inflammatory responses and suppression of odontoblastic properties of KN-3 cells through direct inhibition of LPS [64].

An interesting research concerning ozone was connected with RIT. Regenerative injection therapy (RIT), also known as proliferative therapy, has been used for over 30 years in the USA in patients with spinal and peripheral joint and ligamentous pathologies [38]. It involves the injection of mildly irritating medications onto ligaments and tendons, most commonly at origins and insertions. These injections cause a mild inflammatory response which "turns on" the normal healing process and results in the regeneration of these structures. At the same time they strengthen and become less sensitive to pain through a combination of neurolysis of small nerve fibers (C-fibers) and increased stability of the underlying structures.

Oxygen/ozone therapy is a well established complementary therapy practiced in many European countries. The ozone dissolves in body fluids and immediately reacts with biomolecules generating messengers responsible for biological and therapeutic activities. This results in an anti inflammatory response, which also results in a similar trophic reaction to that of RIT. It is logical to expect that combining these two modalities would result in enhanced healing and therefore improved clinical outcomes. Oxygen/ozone therapy, accomplished by autohemotherapy (AHT), is performed by either administering ozonated blood intravenously (Major AHT) or via intramuscular route (Minor AHT).

These procedures result in stimulation of the immune and healing systems. Our concept is that the local injection of this activated blood injected directly to the ligamentous areas that are also being treated with RIT will act as a direct stimulation to the healing process. In addition, combining this with intravenous major AHT should stimulate the immune system to augment and support this process. RIT and oxygen/ozone therapy have been extensively studied separately. In our opinion this way can be effectively used in many clinical situations in dental patology, for example in patients suffering from chronic artroses of temporo-mandibular joints and other disorders.

Promising is the use of ozone in combination with other active compounds. For example, the combination of ozone with perftoran topically gave a pronounced positive effect of a sharp decline in the prevalence and intensity of the inflammatory infiltrate. As a result of activation of reparative osteogenesis was an intensive formation of bone tissue, which was accompanied by a rapid decrease in the size of the abnormality [36].

Effective is the use of ozone for the prevention of inflammatory complications after surgery in dental surgery (for example, osteosynthesis). Especially, this method is shown in the case of heavy contamination bone wound or oral microflora in the case of a heavy patient's general condition [49].

Ozone can also be potentially used in such important field of dentistry as oral oncology [72]. Tumor hypoxia and ischemia are known to limit treatment efficacy and, hence, the alleviation of such a predisposition to poorer treatment outcome is seen as beneficial. Ozonetherapy can produce an improvement in blood flow and oxygenation in some tissues and although these findings need to be viewed with caution because of the limited number of patients enrolled, ozonetherapy appears to have had some positive effect during the treatment of patients with advanced H&N tumors. The potential usefulness of ozonetherapy as an adjuvant in chemo–radiotherapy for these tumors warrants further investigation. In appropriate concentrations, this technique leads to a transient oxidative stress that can stimulate blood antioxidants by up-regulation. This mechanism has been ascribed to ozone therapy's protection against free radical damage of heart, and prevention of renal and hepatic disorders. Hemolysis of <2.5% and an acceptable level of lipid peroxide formation has been described in autohemotransfusion at O_3/O_2 concentrations of 60 µg/ml. In the course of ozone therapy by autohemotransfusion, ozone, *per se*, does not enter the organism, and its effects are mediated by rapid (a matter of seconds) oxidation of blood components in the transfusion recipient. The oxidized molecules and the specific antioxidant generated would vary according to the levels of ozone therapy. The vascular effect of ozonated blood transfusion is explained by an increase of malonyldialdehyde and lipid peroxidation leading to leading to activation of the hexose monophosphate shunt with an increased production of 2,3-diphosphoglycerate in erythrocytes. This results in a displacement of the oxyhemoglobin dissociation curve to the right and an increase in the release of oxygen to the tissues. A pH decrease in erythrocytes may also shift the oxyhemoglobin dissociation curve to the right (Bohr effect) without modification of 2,3-diphosphoglycerate. Furthermore, a charge modification in red cell membranes results in an improvement in membrane flexibility and a decrease in blood viscosity and resistance. Overall, ozone therapy decreased the percentage of values ≤10 and ≤5 mmHg at each measurement time-point. However, no increase was observed in tumor pO_2, as has been reported in an animal study. In the present study, the oxygenation decreased in tumors with pO_2 concentrations above the median. Based on the oxygen radio-sensitivity curve, it can be inferred that this is not of clinical relevance in well-oxygenated tumors. However, in tumors with baseline pO_2 below the median, i.e. tumors in which the radio-resistance could increase in relation to this 'adverse' value, ozone therapy actually increased the tumor pO_2. This effect is similar to that observed by us in anterior tibialis muscle tissues following the administration of ozone therapy. The mechanisms underlying this effect in tumors have yet to be defined. Based on previously described effects, we hypothesize that the inverse correlation between initial oxygenation and ΔpO_2 in tumors and tissues during ozone therapy is secondary to blood flow redistribution, i.e., a drop in blood flow in well-oxygenated tissues in favor of less well-oxygenated tissues. Tumor vessels have structural and functional abnormalities with decreased or absent auto-regulatory mechanisms. Hence, an improvement in blood rheologic parameters, as described by other authors, could play an important role in the effect of ozone therapy in high-resistance systems such as in tumors; this could apply to at least the areas of the tumor that are most hypoxic. Congruent with this concept is the improvement we observed with ozone therapy in patients with lower hemoglobin levels and, as a consequence, with lower blood viscosity. This vascular effect is further supported by our preliminary studies with Doppler techniques, indicating a lasting blood flow increase following three alternating ozone therapy sessions (B. Clavo, personal communication). Tumor hypoxia predisposes to a physiologic selection of tumor cells with decreased apoptotic potential, which results in resistance to radiotherapy and chemotherapy, higher angiogenesis and a more aggressive tumor potential. If ozone therapy successfully decreases tumor hypoxia in some patients, it could be useful as an adjuvant in the treatment of these patients by improving tumor oxygenation, by reducing radio-resistance and improving local control. Survival could be improved by decreasing tumor hypoxia, as shown by Overgaard's meta-analyses. The results of the present study indicate that tumor pO_2 modification could support the anecdotal clinical reports of an improved effect of radiotherapy in advanced tumors when ozone therapy is included in the schedule [22]. In conclusion, many aspects regarding the bio-medical application of ozone therapy remain unexplored. In the present prospective study, the effect of ozone therapy on human tumor pO_2 has been measured using the polarographic probe technique, and the results indicate that ozone therapy could increase oxygenation in the most hypoxic tumors. This suggests the potential use of this therapy as adjuvant in chemo-radiotherapy schedules, and would warrant further investigation.

Estrela et al. studied antimicrobial effects of ozonated water, gaseous ozone and antiseptic agents (2.5 % hypochlorite and 2 % chlorhexidine) in infected human dental root canals. All these substances had no antibacterial effect against Enterococcus faecalis over a 20 minute contact time in the infected root canals.

Thanomsub et al. tested the effects of ozone treatment on cell growth and ultrastructural changes in bacteria (Escherichia coli, Salmonella sp., Staphylococcus aureus and Bacillus subtilis). It was discovered that ozone at 0.167 mg/min/l can be used to sterilize water, which is contaminated with up to 105 mg/ml bacteria within 30 minutes. Destroying of bacterial cell membrane was observed, subsequently producing intercellular leakage and eventually causing cell lysis.

Kronusova used ozone in following cases: prevention of dental caries in fissures of the first permanent molars in children, application of ozone in prepared cavity, after tooth extraction, in case of postextractional complications, in patients with chronic gingivitis, periodontitis and periodontal abscesses, herpes labialis,
purulent periodontitis, dentition difficilis etc. Almost all patients with gingivitis showed subjective and objective improvement of their status, as well as patients with periodontal abscess, where no exudation was observed. Application of ozone after tooth extraction was found also

quite useful – only 10 % of patients suffered from such complication as alveolitis sicca, but even in these cases the clinical course was shorter and more moderate.

Cosmetic dentists should take note that we have also used ozone to whiten teeth. Ozone sends activated oxygen below the enamel surface, much the same way as the dental bleaches. It is very important that vital bleaching with ozone to reduce the concentration of hydrogen peroxide 15%. This eliminates such a problem as hyperesthesia symptom hard tooth tissues while maintaining high bleaching ability [53].

It is important to note that there is little data on the application of ozone in prosthetic dentistry. In general, the well-known works are devoted to cleaning dentures using a variety of ozonated solutions [65]. Over time, removable dentures tend to become unsanitary and emit unpleasant odors, and oral mucosa sometimes becomes inflamed or denture stomatitis is caused by denture plaque. The combination of ozonated water and ultrasonication had a strong effect on the viability of C. albicans adhering to the acrylic resin plates [3]. Recently, various cleaning products designed to keep removable dentures sanitary have appeared on the market. It is known that denture plaque is mainly composed of Candida albicans (C. albicans), and that ozone seems to inhibit these micro-organisms. Accordingly, a denture cleaner using ozone bubbles (ozone concentration of about 10 ppm) was considered as clinically appropriate because of its strong disinfecting and deodorizing power, and high biological safeness. The effectiveness of this cleaner against C. albicans was investigated using. Results showed that C.

albicans decreased to about 1/10 after 30 min and to 1/10(3) after 60 min [59].

Nevertheless using of ozone in dental practice, in particular prosthodontics, is, in our opinion, insufficiently. Many aspects of using ozonetherapy are not completely discovered, that's why the purpose of our study was to show the effectiveness of local ozonetherapy using the example of its application among patients with removable dentures.

45 patients (25 female and 20 male) with total defects of dentitions were examined. Its important to say that most of them were negatively disposed to removable dentures and didn't believe that they could adaptate to these constructions. All patients were divided into two groups: the first one included patients who used ozonated olive oil for applications on the prosthetic filed for 2 weeks after prosthetics; patients from the second group didn't receive any additional treatment. Comprehensive survey of patients conducted as before prosthetic so as for 3 months after.

Ozonated olive oil was produced using the "Medozons BM-01" device (Medozons, The Russian Federation) by means of its ozonation with the following parameters: the time of ozonation of 100 ml of oil with the concentration of ozone in ozone-air mixture 20 mg/ml was 20 minutes. In this form the ozone has long anti-inflammatory, antiseptic activity, stimulates regeneration and metabolism in oral mucosa.

In addition to standard clinical examination the evaluation of hygienic condition of removable dentures was made using the method of Ambjornsen.

Research of salivation included the determination of its speed, viscosity an pH of a saliva.

Cytological research of the oral mucosa included evaluation of indexes of differentiation and keratinization of epithelial cells.

Mucosal resistance was determined using the reaction of absorption of microorganisms by epithelial cells.

Microbiological study included quantitive and qualitive evaluation of oral microflora using the MicroScan Walk Away 40+ (Siemens, USA).

Also all patients completed special questionnaires to determine the speed of their adaptation to removable laminar dentures.

Analysis of the results showed that hygienic condition of removable dentures of patients with no additional treatment degraded over time (from 3,2±0,26 to 5,5±0,24). In a case of using ozone because of its cleaning effect this parameter was much better (1,9±0,48), but also rised to 3 month. Nevertheless we consider this effect rather important in the initial period of using dentures.

Using removable dentures among most patients led to acceleration of salivation and also decreasing the viscosity of saliva for several weeks after prosthetics. But these parameters returned to original meanings to 3 month after it.

There was interesting difference in the levels of pH of saliva between patients of selected groups: 7,13±0,17 – in ozonetherapy group and 6,72±0,32 in comparison group (14 day after prosthetics). It could be explained by positive action of ozone on the epithelial cells of saliva glands and microflora of oral cavity.

Microbiological research showed that absence of treatment led to growth of quantity of microorganism which were found before prosthetics, and also appearance of new ones during 3 months of research. In ozonetherapy group these parameters saved on original level. These results could be explained by long antiseptic effect of ozonized oil, that on the one hand led to growth suppression of microflora, but on the over hand didn't lead to dysbiosis in oral cavity.

Cytological indexes were also rather different between groups: there was determined the acceleration of regeneration (growth of indexes of differentiation and keratinization of epithelial cells) among patients used local ozonetherapy (Fig. 1). In the comparison group the results were much lower (negative action of removable dentures).

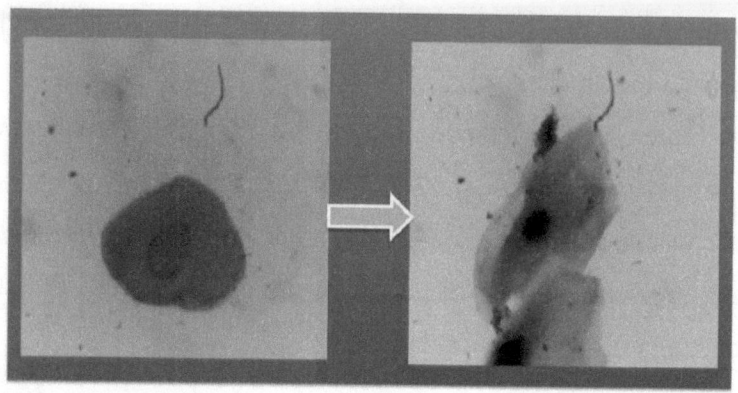

Fig. 1. [Before treatment] of differentiation [After ozonetherapy] after ozonetherapy

Especially important that the resistance of oral mucosa after treatment was much higher: the reaction of absorption of microorganisms by epithelial cells showed significant growth even comparatively meanings before prosthetics (Fig. 2). It could be explained as by improvement of condition of epithelial cells so as reduction of activity of oral microflora.

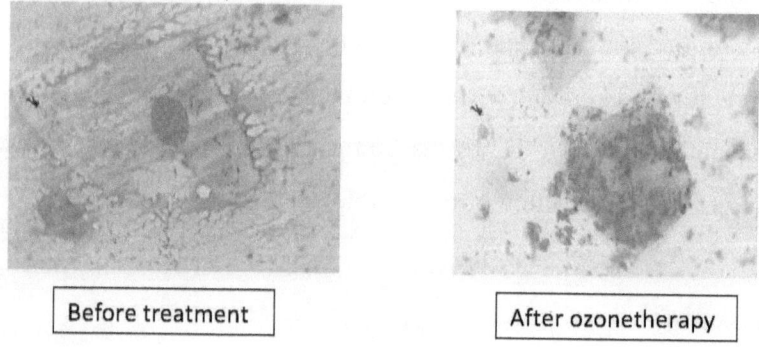

Fig. 2. The increasing of ability of epithelial cells to absorb microorganisms

Analysis of questionnaires showed the reduction of courses of adaptation of elderly patients to complete removable dentures (21,4±2,2 – in ozonetherapy group, 27,2±3,4 – with no additional treatment).

Our research showed high effectiveness of local ozonetherapy among patients used complete removable dentures: the improvement of hygienic condition of dentures, oral mucosa, saving of normal condition of oral microflora and reduction of courses of adaptation of patients to removable dentures.

In patients with partial removable dentures analysis of the results showed that status of oral hygiene of patients didn't significantly differ before prosthetics. But after 14 days the level of plaque index in ozonetherapy group was much lower (1,28±0,12 points), than of patients who didn't receive additional treatment (2,31±0,24 points). This difference was saved to the end of research.

As a result of bad oral hygiene and irritative action of removable laminar dentures gingival index (index PMA) was very high among patients of second group. Using of ozone led to significant reduction of inflammation of gums in the first group, and also very important that these results were determined at the end of study (Fig. 3).

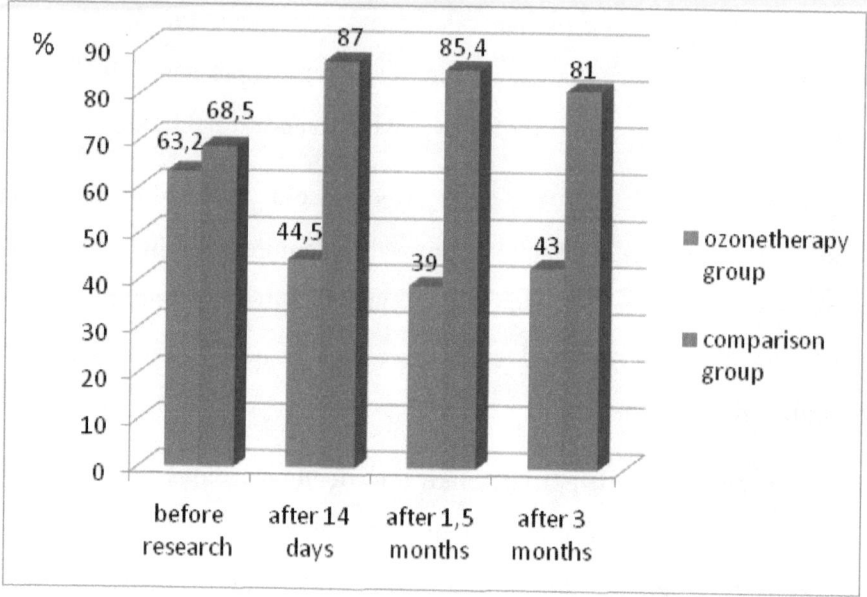

Fig 3. Dynamics of gingival index (PMA) of patients with removable partial laminar dentures

Research of the SBI showed the same result. There was significant reduction of the bleeding index after local ozonetherapy and its rise in group with no additional treatment. These results were agreed to the materials from previous research [5].

One of the possible factors that could explain these results was the influence of ozone therapy on oral microflora, that was proved as clinically (according to reduction of demineralization activity of dental plaque from 1,83±0,32 to 1,3±0,27 among patients used ozonated oil to the 14 day after beginning of the study) such as in laboratories (there was a tendency of saving of normal condition of oral microflora among patients in first group and its growth among patients from the second one).

Study of salivation didn't show any significant results. Among most of patients from both groups salivation was accelerated after prosthetics during 14 days with the reduction of a viscosity of saliva that could be explained by irritative action of removable dentures. But these parameters returned to the original meanings to 3 month. There was interesting difference between the pH-levels of saliva among selected groups (its level was higher among patients used local ozone therapy), that could be explained by lower activity of inflammatory process and microflora in oral cavity (Fig. 4).

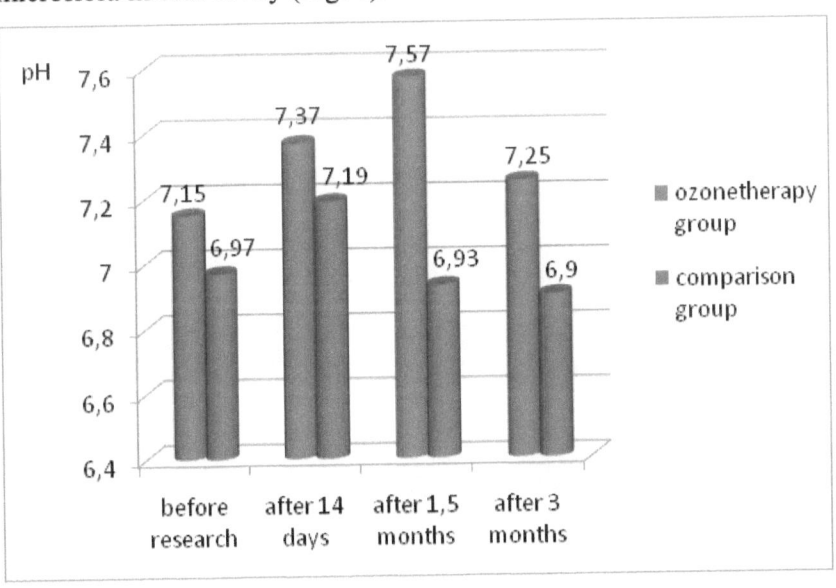

Fig 4. Dynamics of pH of saliva of patients used removable partial laminar dentures

Analysis of questionnaires showed the reduction of courses of adaptation to removable laminar dentures in case of using local ozone therapy indifferently of the sizes of dentition defects (16,5±5,3 days among patients used ozone and 21,4±2,4 days – with no additional treatment).

So, local ozone therapy promotes the reduction of the course of adaptation of elderly patients to partial removable laminar dentures on account of improvement of oral hygiene, condition of periodontal tissues and activity of oral microflora.

We are sure that these and many other effects of ozone can be effectively used in dental practice in different clinical situations.

Conclusion.

In contrast with traditional medicine modalities such as antibiotics and disinfectants, ozone therapy is quite economical; it will markedly reduce both medical cost and invalidity. Dentistry is varying with induction of modern science to practice dentistry. The ozone therapy has been more beneficial than present conventional therapeutic modalities that follow a minimally invasive and conservative application to dental treatment. The exposition of molecular mechanisms of ozone further benefits practical function in dentistry. Treating patients with ozone therapy lessens the treatment time with an immense deal of variation and it eradicates the bacterial count more specifically. The treatment is painless and increases the patients' tolerability and fulfillment with minimal adverse effects. Contraindications of this controversial method should not be forgotten.

The future of ozone therapy must focus on the establishment of safe and well-defined parameters in accordance with randomized, controlled trials to determine the precise indications and guidelines in order to treat various medical and dental pathologies. Scientific support, as suggested by demonstrated studies, for ozone therapy presents a potential for an atraumatic, biologically-based treatment for conditions encountered in dental practice.

References

1. Alekhine SP, Shcherbatyuk T. Ozone: Clinical and Experimental Aspects / / N. Novgorod: Publishing House of the "Letter". - 2003. - 240.

2. Agrillo A., Sassano P., Rinna C. and others. Ozone therapy in extractive surgery on patients treated with bisphosphonates// The journal of craniofacial surgery. – 2007. - №5. – P. 1068-1070.

3. Arita M. and others. Microbicidal efficacy of ozonated water against candida albicans adhearing to acrylic denture plates// Oral microbiology and immunology. – 2005. - №4. – P. 206-210.

4. Arslan S. and others. Effects of different cavity desinfectants on share bond strength of a silorane-based resin composite// The journal of contemporary dental practise. – 2011. - №4. – P. 279-286.

5. Atabeck D., Oztas N. Effectiveness of ozone with or without additional use of remineralising solutions on non-cavitated fissure carious lesions in permanent molars// European journal of dentistry. – 2011. - №4. – P. 393-399.

6. Alyasova AV Kontorshikova KN, Shahs BG Ozone technology in the treatment of malignant tumors / / N. Novgorod: Acad NizhGMA. - 2006. - 204 p.

7. Azarpazhooh A., Limeback H. The application of ozone in dentistry: a systematic review of literature// Journal of dentistry. – 2008. - №2. – P. 104-116.

8. Azarpazhooh A., Limeback H., Lawrence H. P., Fillery E. D. Evaluating the effect of an ozone delivery system on the reversal of

dentin hypersensibility: a randomized, double-blinded clinical trial// Journal of endodontics. – 2009. - №1. – P. 1-9.

9. Baysan A., Lynch E. The use of ozone in dentistry and medicine. Part 2. Ozone and root caries// Primary dental care. – 2006. - №1. – P. 37-41.

10. Baysan A., Lynch E. The use of ozone in dentistry and medicine// Primary dental care. – 2005. - №2. – P. 47-52.

11. Baysan A., Lynch E. Effect of ozone on the oral microbiota and clinical severiry of primary root caries// American Journal of Dentistry. – 2004. - №1. – P. 56-60.

12. Beck E. G., Wasser. G., Viebahn-Hansler. The current status of ozone therapy. Empirical develompent and future research// Forch Komplementared. – 1998. - №5. – P. 61-75.

13. Bezirtzoglou E., Cretoiu S. M. and others. A quantitive approach to the effectiveness of ozone against microbiota organisms colonizing toothbrushes// Journal of dentistry. – 2008. - №8. – P. 600-605.

14. Bezrukov IV, Grudyanov AI use of medical ozone in dentistry / / Dentistry. - 2001. - № 2. - S. 61-63.

15. Bezrukov IV, Petrukhina NB Ozone therapy in periodontal practice / / Moscow Medical News Agency. - 2008. - 88 p.

16. Bezrukov IV, Petrukhina NB, NA Dmitriev, Snegiryov MV Application of medical ozone in endodontic practice (preliminary results of microbiological testing) / / Dentistry. - 2008. - № 6. - S. 24-26.

17. Bocci V. Biological and clinical effects of ozone. Has ozone therapy a future in medicine?// British Journal of Biomedical Science. – 1999. - №56. – P. 270-279.

18. Bocci V. Ozone as Janus: this controversial gas can be either toxic or medically useful// Mediators of inflamation. – 2004. - № 13 (1). – P. 3-11.

19. Bocci V., Borelli E., Travagli V., Zanardi I. The ozone paradox: ozone is a strong oxidant as well as a medical drug// Medicinal research reviews. – 2009. - №4. – P. 646-682.

20. Bojar W., Czarnecka B., Prylinski M., Walory J. Shear bond strength of epoxy resin-based endodontic sealers to bovine dentine after ozone application// Acta of bioengineering and biomechanics. – 2009. - №3. – P. 41-45.

21. Case P. D., Bird P. S. and others. Treatment of root canal biofilms of enterococcus faecalis with ozone gas and passive ultrasound activation// Journal of endodontics. – 2012. - №4. - P. 523-526.

22. Clavo B., Peres J., and others. Ozone Therapy for Tumor Oxygenation: a Pilot Study// Evid Based Complement Alternat Med. - 2004. - №1. – P. 93–98.

23. Dahnhardt J. E., Gygax M., Martignoni B., Suter P., Lussi A. Treating sensitive cervical areas with ozone. A prospective controlled clinical trial// American journal of dentistry. – 2008. - №2. – P. 74-76.

24. Dahnhardt J. E., Jaeggi T., Lussi A. Treating open carious lesions in anxious children with ozone. A prospective controlled clinical study// American journal of dentistry. – 2006. - №5. – P. 267-270.

25. Dmitrieva, LA, Tebloeva L., Gurevich, IG, Zoloeva ZE, Nikolaeva, EI Features changes in the microflora of the periodontal pocket using ozone therapy / / Periodontology. - 2004. - № 4 (33). - Pp. 20-24.

26. Duggal M. S., Nikolopoulou A., Tahmassebi J. F. The additional effect of ozone in combination with adjunct remineralisation products in inhibition of deminaralisation of the dental hard tissues in situ// Journal of dentistry. – 2012. –

27. Dhingra K., Vandana K. L. Management of gingival inflammation in orthodontic patients with ozonated water irrigation – a pilot study// International journal of dental hygiene. – 2011. - №4. – P. 296-302.

28. Dukic W., Dukic O. L., Milardovic S. The influence of healozone on microleakage and fissure penetration of different sealing materials// Collegium antropologicum. – 2009. - №1. – P. 157-162.

29. Dvorak V. Ozon. Vyuziti ozonu ve stomatologii// Progresdent. – 2004. - №3. – C. 8-9.

30. El Hadary A. A., Yassin H. H., and others. Evaluation of the effect of ozonated plant oils an the quality of osteointegration of dental implants under the influence of cyclosporin. A an in vivo study// Journal of oral implantology. – 2011. – №2. – P. 247-257.

31. Filippi A. The influence of ozonized water on the epitelial wound healing process in the oral cavity.

32. Fish OB Comparative evaluation of the effectiveness of non-drug treatment of chronic inflammatory / / Postgraduate Journal of the Volga region. - 2008. - № 3-4. - S. 166-169.

33. Flails LM, Levchenkova NS, Kovalev OV Application Ozone DTA-ozone generator for the treatment of root canals / / Institute of Dentistry. - 2010. - № 3. - S.

34. Frohme H., Rleinert T., Zajicova L. Karies heilen mit HealOzone// Dental Spiegel. – 2003. - №5. – S. 28

88-89.

35. Garcia E. J., Serrano A. P., and others. Influence of ozone gas and ozonated water application to dentin and bonded interfaces on resin-dentin bond strength// The journal of adhesive dentistry. – 2012. - №4. – P. 363-370.

36. Grigoryan, Grigor'yants DA, Guchetl MN Experimental morphological study of the anti-inflammatory action of the complex

applications of ozone-perftoran / / Dentistry. - 2008. - № 2. - P. 4-9.

37. Good M., El K. I., Hussey D. L. Endodontics solutions part 1: a literature review on the use of endodontic lubricants, irrigants and medicaments// Dental update. – 2012. - №4. – P. 239-246

38. Gracer. R. I., Bocci V. Can the combination of localized "proliferative therapy" with "minor ozonated autohemotherapy" restore the natural healing process?// Medical Hypotheses. – 2005. - №65. – P. 752-759.

39. Grootveld M., Silwood C. J., Lynch E. High resolution 1H NMR investigations of the oxidative consumption of salivary biomolecules by ozone: relevance to the therapeutic applications of this agent in clinical dentistry// BioFactors. – 2006. – №1. – P. 5-18.

40. Gursoi H., Cakar G. and others. In vivo evaluation of the effects of different treatment procedures on dentine tubules// Photomedicine and laser surgery. – 2012. - №

41. Gupta G., Mansi B. Ozone therapy in periodontics// Journal of medicine and life. – 2012. - №1. – P. 59-67.

42. Hauser-Gerspach I., Pfaffli-Savtchenko V., Dahnhardt J. E., Meyer J., Lussi A. Comparison of the immediate effects of gaseous ozone and chlorhexidine gel on bacteria in cavitated carious lesions in children in vivo// Clinical Oral Investigations. – 2009. - №3. – P. 287-291.

43. Hauser-Gerspach I., Vadaszan J. Influence of gaseous ozone in peri-implantitis: bactericadal efficacy and cellular response. An in vitro study using titanium and zirconia// Clinical oral investigations. – 2012. - №4. – P. 1049-1059.

44. Holmes J. Clinical reversal of root caries using ozone, double-blind, randomised, controlled 18-month trial// Gerontology. – 2003. - №2. – P. 106-114.

45. Huth K. C., Jakob F. M. Effect of ozone on oral cells compared with established antimicrobials// European journal of oral sciences. – 2006. - №5. – P. 435-440.

46. Huth K. C., Paschos E., Brand K., Hickel R. Effect of ozone on non-cavitated fissure carious lesions in permanent molars. A controlled prospective clinical study// American Journal of Dentistry. – 2005. - №4. – P. 223-228.

47. Huth K. C., Quirling M., Lenzke S. and others. Effectiveness of ozone against periodontal pathogenic microorganisms// European Journal of Oral sciences. – 2011. - №3. – P. 204-210.

48. Huth K. C., Quirling M., Maier S. Effectiveness of ozone against endodotopathogenic microorganisms in a root canal biofilm model// International endodontis journal. – 2009. - №1. – P. 3-13.

49. Inkarbekov JB, Dzhunusova G. The use of ozone for the prevention of inflammatory complications after osteosynthesis of the mandible / / Institute of Dentistry. - 2007. - № 4. - S. 88-89.

50. Johansson E., Andersson-Wenckert I., Hagenbjork-Gustafsson A. and others. Ozone air levels adjacent to a dental ozone gas delivery system// Acta odontologica Scandinavica. – 2007. - №6. – P. 324-330.

51. Kazarina LN, Volozhin AI ozone-and girudoterapiya in treatment glossalgia

52. Knight G. M., McIntyre J. M., Craig G. G. and others. The inability of streptococcus mutans and lactobacillus acidophilus to form a biofilm in vitro on dentine pretreated with ozone// Australian dental journal. – 2008. - №4. – P. 349-353.

53. Krikheli NI Yanushevich OO, Bichikaeva ZA Experience of using ozone for bleaching vital teeth / / Dentistry for all. - 2009. - № 2. - P. 4-6.

54. Kronenberg O., Lussi A., Ruf S. Preventive effect of ozone on the development of white spot lesions during multibracket appliance therapy// The angle ortodontist. – 2009. - №1. – P. 64-69.

55. Lunin VV Healing ozone / / Science in Russia. - 2006. - № 4. - S. 17-21.

56. Maslennikov, OV, Kontorshikova KN Practical ozone therapy. Manual / / N. Novgorod: Publishing House of the "Vector TiS." - 2003. - 52.

57. Maslennikov, OV, Kontorshikova KN, fungal IA Guide to ozone therapy / / N. Novgorod: Publishing House of the "Vector-Tees." - 2008. - 326 p.

58. Minenkov AA Filimonov, RM, Pokrovsky VI Basic principles and tactics of ozone therapy / / Moscow Medozon. - 2000. -

59. Murakami H., Sakuma S. and others Desinfection of removable dentures using ozone// Dental materials journal. – 1996. - №2. – P. 220-225.

60. Nagayoshi M., Fukuizumi T., Kitamura C. and others. Efficacy of ozone on survival and permeability of oral microorganisms// Oral microbiology and immunology. – 2004. - №4. – P. 240-246.

61. Nagayoshi M., Kitamura C., Fukuizumi T., Nishihara T., Terashita M. Antimicrobal effect of ozonated water on bacteria invading dentinal tubules// Journal of endodontics. – 2004. - №11. – P. 78-81

62. Noetzel J. and others. Efficacy of calcium hydroxide, ErYAG laser or gaseous ozone against Enterococcus faecalis in root canals// American journal of dentistry. – 2009. - №1. – P. 14-18.

63. Nogales C. G., Ferrari P. H., Kantorovich E. O., Lage-Marques J. L. Ozone therapy in medicine and dentistry// The journal of contemporary dental practise. – 2008. - №4. – P. 75-84.

64. Noguchi F., Kitamura C.and others. Ozonated water improves lipopolysaccharide-induced responses of an odontoblast-like cell time// Journal of endodontics. – 2009. - №5. – P. 668-672.

65. Oizumi M., Suzuki T., Uchida M. and others. In vitro testing af a denture cleaning method using ozone// Journal of medical and dental science. – 1998. - №2. – P. 135-139.

66. Paolo N., Bocci V., Gaggiotti E. Ozone therapy (editorial review)// The International Journal of Artificial Organs. – 2004. - №3. – P. 168-175.

67. Polydorou O., Halili A., Wittmer A. and others. The antibacterial effect of gas ozone after 2 months of in vitro evaluation// Clinical oral investigations. – 2012. - №2. – P. 545-550.

68. Raafat Abdelaziz R., Mossalam R. S., Yousry M. M. Tubular occlusion of simulated hypersensitive dentine by the combined use of ozone end desensitizing agents// Acta odontologica Scandinavica. – 2011. - №6. – P. 395-400.

69. Sadatullah S., Mohsmed N. H., Razak F. A. The antimicrobal effect of 0,1 ppm ozonated water on 24-hour plaque microorganisms in situ// Brasilian oral research. – 2012. - №2. – P. 126-131.

70. Saini R. Ozone therapy in dentistry: a stratagic review// Journal of natural Science, biology and medicine. – 2011. - №2. – P. 151-153.

71. Seidler V., Linetskiy I. and others. Ozone and its usage in general medicine and dentistry. A review article// Prague medical report. – 2008. - №1. – P. 5-13.

72. Shcherbatyuk T. The current state of ozone therapy in medicine. Prospects for application in oncology // STM. - 2010. - № 1. - S. 99-106.

73. Short NG, Scout O. Dmitriev, VV Effect of ozone on microbial haraktirestiki oral fluid of patients with fractures of the mandible // Dentistry. - 2000. - № 2. - S. 20-21.

74. Silveira A. M., Lopes H. P., Siqueira J. F. and others. Periradicular repair after two-visit endodontic treatment using two different intracanal medications compared to single visit endodontic treatment// Brasilian dental Journal. – 2007. - №4. – P. 299-304.

75. Skurska A., Pietruska M. D., Paniczko-Drezek A. and others. Evaluation of the influence of ozonetherapy on the clinical parameters and MMP levels in patients with chronic and aggressive periodontitis// Advances in medical sciences. – 2010. - №2. – P. 297-307.

76. Stoll R., Venne L. and others. The disinfecting effect of ozonized oxygen in an infected root canal: an in vitro study// Quintessence international. – 2008. - №3. – P.231-236.

77. Stopka P. Ozon. Fyzikalni, chemicke, biologicke vlastnosti a ucinky, vyskut v prirode, detekce, manipulace// Progressdent. – 2003. - №6. – S. 8-11.

78. Stubinger S., Sader R., Filippi A. The use of ozone in dentistry and maxillofacial surgery: a review// Quintessence international. – 2006. - №5. – P. 353-359.

79. Tessier J., Rodriguez P. N., and others. The use of ozone to lighten teeth. An experimental study// Acta odontologica latinoamericana. – 2010. - №2. – P. 84-89.

80. Travagli V., Zanardi I., Valacchi G., Bocci V// Ozone and ozonated oil in skin diseases: a review// Mediators inflammation. – 2010.

81. Wang R. R., Shang G. W. and others. The disinfecting effect of ozone on four kinds of bacteria// Shanghai journal of stomatology. – 2008. - №1. – P. 92-95.

82. Wilczynska-Borawska M., and othres. Ozone in dentistry: microbilogical effects of gas action depending on the method and the time of application using the ozonytron device. Experimental study// Annales Academiae Medicae Stetinensis. – 2011. – №2. – P. 99-103.

83. Zaura E., Buijs M. J., Cate J. M. Effect of ozone and sodium hypochlorite on caries-like lesions in dentine// Caries Research. – 2007. - №6. – P489-492.

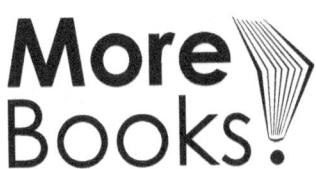
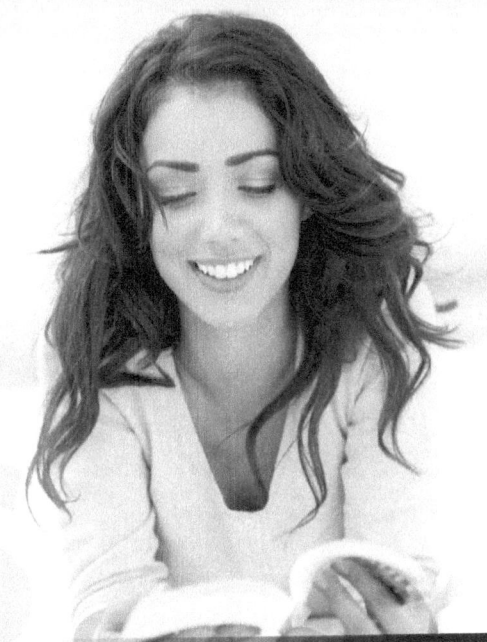

I want morebooks!

Buy your books fast and straightforward online - at one of the world's fastest growing online book stores! Environmentally sound due to Print-on-Demand technologies.

Buy your books online at

www.get-morebooks.com

Kaufen Sie Ihre Bücher schnell und unkompliziert online – auf einer der am schnellsten wachsenden Buchhandelsplattformen weltweit! Dank Print-On-Demand umwelt- und ressourcenschonend produziert.

Bücher schneller online kaufen

www.morebooks.de

OmniScriptum Marketing DEU GmbH
Heinrich-Böcking-Str. 6-8
D - 66121 Saarbrücken

Telefax: +49 681 93 81 567-9

info@omniscriptum.de
www.omniscriptum.com

www.ingramcontent.com/pod-product-compliance
Lightning Source LLC
Chambersburg PA
CBHW031545210526
45464CB00003B/1160